Fitness Routines for Busy Moms

Quick and Efficient

Harmony Royce

DEDICATION

To everyone who strives for inner serenity, harmony, and wellbeing despite all of life's challenges. This book offers courage, resiliency, and inspiration for personal development. As you travel along the path to a happy and fulfilled life, I hope that these words serve as a beacon for you.

CONTENTS

ACKNOWLEDGMENTS

The knowledge, support, and inspiration of numerous people and sources came together to create this book. I sincerely thank everyone who contributed to its creation.

I would like to thank my family and friends for their unwavering support, tolerance, and understanding during this endeavor. Your support has served as both my motivation and compass during difficult and creative moments.

I am indebted to the mental health professionals whose expertise and dedication contributed to the formation of this book's content. Your commitment to helping individuals navigate the complexities of the mind is very admirable.

As they set out on this path of self-discovery and advancement, I am appreciative of the readers who have trusted me with their time and attention. My sincere hope is that the wisdom contained inside these pages resonates with you and motivates you to create a resilient, balanced, and fulfilling life.

Finally, I would like to thank the entire team at SmartWave Research Group for their enthusiasm, guidance, and experience in making this project a success.

With profound appreciation.

DISCLAIMER

This book's content is meant solely for educational reasons; it is not meant to take the place of expert medical advice, diagnosis, or treatment. Regarding any specific health issues or inquiries, readers should speak with licensed healthcare providers. The use of the information in this book may have unfavorable effects, consequences, or outcomes for which the author and publisher disclaim all liability. Since each person's health situation is different, what works for one person might not work for another. It is recommended that readers exercise caution and good judgment when applying any information found in this book to their personal situations.

CHAPTER 1

WHY BUSY MOMS SHOULD BE FIT

1.1 The Strength of Movement: Elevate Your Mood and Energy

Consider that you are a battery, much like the ones that power your devices or toys. You can run, play, think, and do everything you enjoy with the support of this battery. However, if you use it more, the battery may run out and you'll feel drained and irritable. Exercise and movement are like a specific charger for this battery. Mothers who exercise their bodies are able to replenish their energy reserves and do tasks with greater vigor.

Additionally, exercise produces "endorphins" in the brain. Endorphins resemble little happiness enhancers. Moms experience happiness and relaxation when they exercise because of these endorphins. Therefore, moving about benefits the mind as much as the body!

1.2 Strengthening Yourself for Daily Tasks

Have you ever witnessed your mother picking you up for a bear hug or hauling heavy grocery bags? Strength is needed for these tasks. Moms may perform these daily tasks more effortlessly when they have stronger muscles from exercise. Imagine your muscles as the internal superheroes in your body. Moms build their superhero muscles through exercise, which increases their strength and power.

For instance, your mother can carry all those supermarket bags without becoming fatigued when she strengthens her arms with push-ups and weightlifting. She will find it easier to run around in the park with you if you exercise her legs with squats and running. Moms can manage their hectic days and feel less exhausted by strengthening themselves.

1.3 Setting Your Own Needs First: Mental and Physical Health

Mothers serve as the family's captains, directing everyone and ensuring that everything goes without a hitch. However, there are instances when people get so preoccupied with looking after everyone else that they neglect themselves. Moms who prioritize fitness are taking the time to take care of their own physical and mental well-being.

Moms who exercise on a regular basis treat themselves like wonderful treats. They feel better, can think more clearly, and can unwind thanks to it. This "me-time" is crucial since a contented mother is better able to care for her family. Maternity mothers require their own time to exercise and feel well, just as you do.

1.4 Realistic Goal-Setting: Minor Actions, Major Impact

Recall the day you acquired your bike riding skills. You didn't start off riding incredibly quickly or performing spectacular stunts. You started out little, learning how to peddle and balance. Goal-setting for fitness functions similarly. Mothers do not have to immediately run a marathon. They might begin with modest, doable objectives and work their way up from there.

A mother might set out to walk for ten minutes a day, for instance. She might try jogging or walking for twenty minutes if she gets acclimated to it. Over time, these little actions add up to produce significant outcomes. Similar to assembling Lego bricks, one component at a time can result in an incredible creation!

Fitness is crucial for working mothers because it increases their energy, strengthens their bodies for everyday chores, supports their mental and physical well-being, and demonstrates to them that even tiny actions may have a large impact. Therefore, encourage your mother when you see her working out because she's doing great for the family as a whole!

CHAPTER 2

BUSY MOMS' TIME MANAGEMENT TRICKS

2.1 Planning Exercises: Discover Your Fit for the Day

Consider your mother's day as a massive riddle. She needs to juggle work, taking care of you, cooking, cleaning, and possibly even a little self-time. Exercise is one of the key components. However, deciding where to put it might be challenging!

Mothers are able to identify small windows of time during the day that are most productive for them. Perhaps it's right after you go to bed, right before everyone else wakes up, or early in the morning when you nap. Workouts don't have to be lengthy. A little 15 to 20 minutes can have a significant impact. It's similar to figuring out where to put a puzzle piece to finish an image!

2.2 Including the Family: Group Exercises (or Side-by-Side Exercises)

Making exercise a family activity can make it more enjoyable. Imagine running a race in the backyard or performing jumping jacks together. Moms may make exercise time enjoyable for the entire family by including everyone in the routine.

You could go for a bike ride or a walk with your mother, for instance. Alternatively, she may work out while you play close by. It's similar to having an encouraging workout partner. It also teaches everyone the value and enjoyment of remaining active.

2.3 Fast Exercises to Do While You Wait: Increase Downtime

Consider all the times you have to wait for things: you have to wait for the laundry to be finished, for dinner to be ready, or for you to get ready for school. Moms can sneak in brief workouts during these little moments of relaxation.

For example, your mom may perform some lunges or squats in the kitchen as she waits for the water to boil. She might circle the field if she's waiting for your soccer practice to end. Similar to accumulating spare change in a piggy bank, these little exercises add up. Every little bit matters!

2.4 Batching Errands: Combine Daily Tasks with More Movement

Errands are all the tiny things that mothers have to do, such as going to the bank, grocery shopping, and mail pickup. Mothers can "batch" these tasks rather than completing them one at a time. This entails running multiple errands in a single trip, which expedites the day and increases movement.

Your mother might, for instance, park further away from the shop and make the extra walk. Alternatively, she could choose to walk rather than use the lift. She can keep active without needing extra time if she finds methods to move more throughout everyday tasks.

Mothers can include exercise into their hectic schedules by planning daytime workouts, getting the family involved in enjoyable activities, leveraging waiting time for brief workouts, and incorporating extra movement into everyday tasks. These time-management tips support mothers in maintaining their well-being and demonstrate that, despite having a busy schedule, it is always possible to prioritize fitness. So, remember that your mother is taking extra care of the family and herself the next time you see her finding time to work out!

CHAPTER 3

Basic Equipment for a Home Gym (Without Going Over Budget)

3.1 Exercises with Bodyweight: Your Own Personal Gym

What do you think? You always carry around a gym! You are the one with the body. You can perform bodyweight exercises with just your body. You may perform them anywhere, in your living room, backyard, or even your bedroom, as they don't require any specialized equipment.

Cool bodyweight workouts to try are planks, jumping jacks, squats, and push-ups. Your arms are used to raise and lower your body during a push-up. Squats are similar to sitting and getting up without the aid of a chair. Jumping jacks involve extending your arms and legs like a star, then bringing them back in. Planks are people who balance on their hands and toes while maintaining a straight body like a plank of wood. Your body becomes fitter and your muscles become stronger with these activities.

3.2 Utilizing Common Household Items as Creative Tools for Fitness

Exercise doesn't necessarily require expensive gear. Take a look around your home; there are a lot of exercise-related items. Here are some suggestions:

1. Bottles of water: They function similarly to weights. Your mother's arms will get stronger from lifting them.
2. Chairs: Ideal for performing exercises such as tricep dips or step-ups. Step-ups involve rising and falling off of a chair. Using the chair, lower and raise your body with your arms to perform tricep dips.
3. Towels: Excellent for stretches. Your mother can extend her arms and legs by holding a towel.

These commonplace objects resemble covert exercise equipment!

3.3 Investing Sensibly: Needed Equipment for at-home Exercise

Investing in a few items of equipment can occasionally improve sessions even further. However, you don't have to spend a lot of cash. The following items are worthwhile obtaining:

1. Yoga Mat: Excellent for providing comfort when performing floor activities.
2. Resistance Bands: These pliable bands have the potential to strengthen muscles. You can select the one that best suits your needs as they are available in a variety of strengths.
3. Dumbbells: To increase the difficulty of an exercise, hold small weights in your hands.

These things are like tiny assistants that make working out more enjoyable and easier. They are reasonably priced and versatile enough for a wide range of exercises.

3.4 Making Use of Online Resources: Accessible Exercise Programs

There are tons of exercise videos and guidelines on the internet, like a treasure trove. Your mom can use a plethora of free internet resources to maintain her fitness. Numerous videos on websites such as YouTube demonstrate various workout programs and exercises. While some videos are lengthier and ideal for longer workouts, some are shorter and ideal for quick workouts.

Free workouts are also available through several fitness applications. To help your mom stick to her exercise schedule and meet her fitness objectives, some of these apps can even create a customized training plan for her.

Building a home gym doesn't have to be expensive. Mothers can exercise with their own bodies, create new routines using everyday objects, purchase a few basic pieces of equipment, and get free workouts online. Keep yourself in shape at home with these simple and enjoyable strategies. Thus, you'll know your mom is utilizing her at-home gym to the fullest in order to maintain her strength and health when you see her working out with a water bottle or watching a training video!

CHAPTER 4

FIT MOMS ON THE GO: HIGH-INTENSITY INTERVAL TRAINING (HIIT)

4.1 Maximize Outcomes in Less Time: The Science of HIIT

Has there ever been a game where the object is to run as quickly as possible, take a breather, and then run again? It bears a lot of similarities to High-Intensity Interval Training (HIIT). With high-intensity interval training (HIIT), you work out for a brief period of time, recover for a little while, and then repeat. It resembles repeatedly running and then strolling.

HIIT is a great form of exercise since it increases heart rate and builds muscle faster than traditional forms of exercise. It's as if moms with limited time have a superpower that helps them stay in shape. According to scientists, high-intensity interval training (HIIT) is superior to longer, slower-paced exercise in terms of burning calories and increasing muscle mass. It's like being extremely productive and finishing a lot of stuff in a short period of time!

4.2 Example HIIT Exercises: Combinations of Strength and Cardio

Now let's apply HIIT using a few entertaining scenarios. Here are a few examples of high-intensity interval training (HIIT) routines that combine cardio (movements that increase heart rate) and strength (movements that strengthen muscles):

Example of HIIT Exercise 1:

1. Jumping Jacks (30 seconds): Leap up, extending your arms and legs in a star-like motion, and then leap back to your standing position.
2. Rest (30 seconds): Breathe deeply and take a moment to regroup.
3. Squats (30 seconds): Bend your knees, lower your body as though seated in an unseen chair, and then raise yourself to a standing position.

4. Relax (30 seconds): Take a moment to unwind.

5. High Knees (30 seconds): While running in place, raise your knees to the maximum extent possible.

6. Recess (30 seconds): Take a deep breath and prepare for the following activity.

7. Push-Ups (30 seconds): Use your hands and toes to lower your body to the floor, then push yourself back up.

Model HIIT Exercise 2:

1. Burpees (30 seconds): Jump up, crouch down, extend your legs into a plank, perform a push-up, and then jump up again.

2. Relax (30 seconds): Let your muscles relax.

3. Lunges (30 seconds): Bend both knees while stepping forward with one foot, then swap legs.

4. Relax (30 seconds): Breathe out.

5. Mountain Climbers (30 seconds): Quickly switch legs while in a plank posture by bringing one knee to your chest.

6. Slumber (30 seconds): Unwind a little.

7. Plank (30 seconds): Balance on your forearms and

toes while maintaining a straight body posture.

8.

9. Even though each workout just lasts a few minutes, it's really effective!

4.3 Tailoring HIIT to Your Degree of Fitness: Begin slowly and advance gradually.

It's acceptable if not everyone can begin with an extremely strenuous workout! You may adjust HIIT to suit any level of fitness. Moms can begin with milder versions of certain exercises and gradually increase their difficulty if they feel too hard.

Moms can perform push-ups on their knees or against a wall, for instance, if standard push-ups are too challenging. Stepping side to side can be substituted for jumping jacks if it becomes too exhausting. The secret is to start off slowly and increase the difficulty of the exercises as the person gains strength and comfort.

4.4 HIIT Motivation: Keep It Fun and Interesting

Exercise motivation might be difficult to maintain, but HIIT can be a lot of fun! Here are some concepts to maintain the suspense:

1. Music: Playing lively music can transform a workout into a dance party.
2. Challenges: Mothers might establish modest objectives, such as increasing their weekly jumping jacks, and acknowledge their accomplishments.
3. Type: Adding a variety of workouts makes things engaging. It could be strength-focused one day and cardio-focused the next.
4. Time with the Family: HIIT may take on the sense of a game when the family is involved. Youngsters can participate, and everyone can encourage one another.

HIIT is an excellent method for working mothers to lose weight quickly. Moms may get the most out of their fitness program by knowing the science behind it, trying out sample routines, adjusting activities to meet their ability, and having fun. You'll know your mother is channeling her inner superhero to maintain her strength and health the next time you catch her working out for a short while.

CHAPTER 5

BUILDING A STRONG AND TONED BODY WITH STRENGTH TRAINING

5.1 Gaining Muscle: Advantages Beyond Looks

Have you ever seen a muscular superhero in real life? They appear strong and prepared to come to our rescue! However, muscles do much more for us than merely give us a robust appearance. Gaining muscle helps moms lift big supermarket bags, carry you more effortlessly, and even prevent injuries to their bodies.

Daily chores are made easier by strong muscles. Think about how much easier it is to push a heavy door open if you are strong! Additionally, muscles maintain the health of your bones and joints by supporting them. And what do you know? Even while you're at rest, your body uses more energy when it has more muscles. It is comparable to having a constantly operating supercharged engine!

5.2 Exercises for Building Bodyweight Strength: Lunges, Squats, and More

To gain muscle, you don't always need expensive equipment. An incredible tool for strength training is your own body. Moms can try these fantastic bodyweight exercises:

1. Squats: Return to standing after assuming the position of an unseen chair. This workout strengthens your lower body and legs.
2. Lunges: Take a step forward, bending both knees; step back and alternate legs. Lunges improve balance and the strength of your legs.
3. Press-Ups: With your hands on the floor, lie on your stomach and raise and lower your body. Push-ups strengthen your chest and arms.
4. Deck: Maintain an erect posture akin to a wooden plank, maintaining your balance on your hands and toes. For your abdominal muscles, planks are fantastic.

By using your body weight, these exercises build muscle. It

is comparable to weightlifting without the use of weights!

5.3   Easy Equipment Strength Training: Using Resistance Bands or Dumbbells

At times, exercising might be enhanced by a little additional assistance. Simple equipment like resistance bands and dumbbells can help muscles develop stronger and more muscular mass. Here's how to apply them:

1. Incredible weights: You can grasp these tiny weights in your hands. Moms can use them for exercises like shoulder presses, which involve pushing the weights above their heads, or bicep curls, which involve lifting the weights to their shoulders. Using dumbbells strengthens your shoulders and arms.

2. Bands of Resistance: You can pull and push these elastic bands to target different muscle groups. Moms can use them for tricep extensions, which involve pulling the band to train the back of the arms, or band squats, in which they stand on the band and hold the handles while squatting.

These are like having unique devices that up the ante on exercising fun and challenging!

5.4 Concentrating on Particular Muscle Groups: Establish a Well-Rounded Schedule

Moms must strengthen every muscle in their body to maintain their balance and strength, just like a superhero needs all of their powers. They can target various muscle groups in the following ways:

1. Arms: Bicep curls and tricep dips are two exercises that target strengthening the arms.
2. Legs: By strengthening the legs, squats, lunges, and step-ups increase leg power.
3. Core (Tummy and Back): To strengthen the core, perform Russian twists, planks, and sit-ups. These muscles guard the back and aid in balance.
4. Chest and Shoulders: Shoulder presses and push-ups target the upper body, enhancing its strength and durability.

Mothers can design a well-rounded workout program that

maintains the strength and health of their entire body by combining various exercises.

Strength training enables mothers to develop the muscles that maintain their bodies healthy and facilitate daily duties. Moms can develop superhuman strength using bodyweight workouts, basic equipment like dumbbells and resistance bands, and a regimen that works every muscle area. Thus, encourage your mother when you see her lifting weights or performing squats since she is working hard to maintain her strength and health for the benefit of the entire family!

CHAPTER 6

HEART-RATE-BOOSTING CARDIO EXERCISES

6.1 Cardio Options for Active Moms: Dancing and Running

The main goals of cardio exercises are to increase heart rate and physical activity. Think of your heart as a very strong engine that requires periodic revving. Cardiovascular workouts support the health and strength of this engine. Even with hectic schedules, moms can engage in cardio in a variety of enjoyable ways.

Mothers may be fond of running. It's a fantastic method to acquire some fresh air and decompress. Others may have a passion for dancing. Workouts turn into dance parties when music is played! Cycling is another activity that may be done outside or at home on a stationary cycle. Cardio exercises like swimming, jump rope, and even brisk walking are excellent choices. The body becomes healthier and the heart becomes stronger with each of these exercises.

6.2 Indoor Cardio Choices: At-Home Exercises

Moms may still work out cardio at home whether it's raining or too cold outside. These indoor aerobic workouts include:

1. Jumping Jacks: Spread your arms and legs like a star, then leap back up to a standing position. It's easy to do and raises heart rate rapidly.
2. Dancing: Turn up the music and circle the living room while dancing. It's exciting and high-energy.
3. Stair Climbing: Using your home's stairs to ascend and descend multiple times is a fantastic exercise.
4. High Knees: While running, raise your knees as high as you can. This workout strengthens the legs and quickens heart rate.
5. Burpees: Begin in a standing posture, then descend into a squat and leap back to a plank position. Next, perform a push-up, leap back to a squat, and leap to stand. It's quite hard, but it works wonders.

There is no particular equipment required for these workouts, and they can be performed at any time. They can be included into moms' schedules anytime they have a few spare minutes.

6.3 Discover Your Neighborhood for Outdoor Cardio Adventures

Going for a cardio workout outside might be an adventure! Moms can take in the fresh air and go exploring in their area. Here are a few possibilities for outdoor cardio:

1. Running or Jogging: Getting your heart rate up can be achieved by jogging or running around the block. It's also pleasant to see various areas of the neighborhood.
2. Cycling: Riding a bike is a great aerobic exercise, whether you go at a quicker rate or take it slowly.
3. Strolling: Running may not always be better for the heart than a vigorous stroll. Moms can go on walks with friends, the dog, or you.
4. Backpacking: Hiking is a great way to combine

nature with cardio if there are trails around. Every time is like a little adventure.

5. Playground Exercise: Moms can work out on the equipment at the playground while their children play. Exercises like swinging, climbing, and even pursuing someone are highly beneficial.

Exercise becomes more enjoyable when done outside rather than feeling like a duty.

6.4 Finding Fun Activities for Cardio: Make Cardio Fun

Having fun with your aerobic exercises is the greatest way to keep up with them. It's simpler to exercise consistently when it seems like playtime. Here are some suggestions to maintain the fun of cardio:

1. Music and Podcasts: While working out, listening to your favorite music or an engaging podcast can help the time pass quickly.
2. Games: Make working out fun. Establish goals, such as the number of jumping jacks one can perform in a

minute.

3. Fun with the Family: Turn it into a family event. Engage in a dance-off, game of tag, or a group bike ride.

4. Variety: Change things up to maintain interest. To avoid monotony, try experimenting with new things every week.

5. Achievements: Establish modest objectives and treat yourself when you meet them. It may be as easy as enjoying a favorite snack or a soothing bath.

Making time for fun activities guarantees that aerobic exercises become an anticipation rather than a source of anxiety.

Cardiovascular exercise is critical to maintaining a robust and healthy heart. There are several options for busy moms, such dancing and running as well as indoor workouts and outdoor excursions. Cardio can be made entertaining by incorporating games, music, and family activities. This can help exercise become a regular part of life. Thus, you should be proud of your mother for keeping herself in good shape when you see her running or bouncing around!

CHAPTER 7

MOBILE FITNESS: ANYWHERE, ANYTIME WORKOUTS

7.1 Playground Equipment for Park Workouts

Imagine transforming a park into an incredibly entertaining gym. Moms can work out while you play in parks with lots of cool equipment. Here are some suggestions:

1. Monkey Bars: Mothers can perform pull-ups using the monkey bars. They raise their bodies by grabbing the bars. Their backs and arms are extremely strong as a result.

2. Increases in Bench: Locate a stable bench and take small steps. Leg muscles benefit greatly from this exercise. Mothers are even capable of holding your hand while you take steps forward and backward together.

3. Swings: Moms can perform lunges or squats close to you as you swing. In addition, they can perform leg

lifts by holding onto the swing.

4. Climbs on Slides: Moms can attempt going up the slide (if it's safe to do so) as an alternative to sliding down. It's enjoyable to strengthen your entire body in this way.

5. Traversing Routes: A lot of parks have trails or walkways. Moms can watch you while they jog or stroll quickly through the park.

Going to the park becomes an enjoyable fitness journey for all when they use the playground equipment for workouts!

7.2 Travel Fitness: Keep Moving During Pleasure or Work Trips

Maintaining a fitness regimen can be challenging for mothers who travel for business or leisure. However, there are several options to be active wherever one is:

1. Workouts in the Hotel Room: Mothers can work out in their hotel room using bodyweight exercises like planks, squats, and push-ups. It's like having a little gym there!

2. Tours by Foot: Walking around a new location is a terrific way to keep active. Moms can get their quota of steps in while taking walks through the city, visiting museums, and taking in the sights.

3. Stair Climbing: Mothers can use the hotel's stairs as a short cardio exercise if they have any. A few trips up and down the stairs can certainly raise your heart rate.

4. Seaside Exercises: Moms can run on the sand, which is more strenuous than running on tarmac and excellent for their legs, if the vacation destination offers a beach. In addition, they can stretch or do yoga while listening to the sound of the waves.

5. Transportable Devices: Moms can pack lightweight exercise equipment in their luggage, such as resistance bands. You may use these bands anywhere to do a range of strength exercises.

Traveling does not imply a vacation from exercise. Try out some fun and novel approaches to staying active.

7.3 Workouts for the Office: Incorporate Movement Throughout the Day

Even mothers who work in offices can fit in a little exercise during the course of their hectic days. Here's how to do it:

1. Desk Exercises: While seated at a desk, mothers can perform basic exercises like shoulder shrugs, desk push-ups, and seated leg lifts. The muscles remain active with these motions.

2. Walking Meetings: Mothers can recommend walking meetings as an alternative to sitting in a conference room. One of the best ways to get some steps in while working is to walk and talk.

3. Stretch Breaks: Mothers are allowed to take a brief pause to stand and stretch once per hour. The body can remain flexible and energetic via stretching.

4. Stair Breaks: Mothers can utilize the stairs in place of the elevator. A few flights alone might provide a beneficial workout.

5. Walks at Lunchtime: Taking a stroll during your lunch break is a great way to get some exercise and

fresh air.

Moms can maintain their energy and activity levels while working by including these little exercises into their daily routine.

7.4 Fun Exercises for Kids: Convert Playtime into Exercise

Including your kids in your workouts during playtime is one of the finest methods for moms to stay in shape. She gets to workout and you both get to enjoy yourselves, so it's a win-win situation. Here are a few lighthearted suggestions:

1. Tag: Tag is a fantastic cardio exercise. Heart rate is raised by running, dodging, and trying to catch each other.

2. Obstacle Course: Construct a miniature obstacle course in a park or backyard. Moms and children can race around cones, crawl under tables, and jump over poles. It feels like a fun race.

3. Party in the Daze: In the living room, turn up some

music and have a dance off. Dancing is a great method to release tension and have fun with others.

4. Sports Activities: Engage in a game of basketball, soccer, or catch. These sports are great for working out your entire body.

Moms and children may practice yoga together by following a kid-friendly yoga video. It promotes flexibility and balance and is calming.

Moms can spend quality time with you and stay in shape by converting playtime into workout time.

Using your surroundings and your creativity will help you stay active while on the go. Mothers may discover easy and enjoyable ways to keep active, whether they're in the park, on the road, at work, or just having fun with their kids. Thus, the next time you catch your mother working out while you're playing, jump in and let's have a great time together!

CHAPTER 8

FUELING YOUR WORKOUTS WITH NUTRITION FOR BUSY MOMS

8.1 Nutritious Food Practices: Fuel Your Body for the Day

Think of your body as the vehicle of a superhero. You must use the proper fuel in it to ensure that it operates quickly and smoothly. Eating a healthy diet is like putting the best fuel in the bodies of busy moms, allowing them to have plenty of energy for everyday activities and workouts.

Eating healthfully entails selecting foods that are beneficial to your body. Here are some dietary recommendations for mothers:

1. Well-Balanced Meals: A variety of fruits, vegetables, whole grains (such brown rice or whole wheat bread), proteins (like chicken, fish, or legumes), and whole grains should be included in each meal. The

body can receive all the nutrients it requires from this mixture.

2. Nutritious Snacks: Moms can eat fruits, almonds, yogurt, or veggies with hummus as a snack instead of grabbing for chips or candies. Energy from these foods comes without a sugar crash.

3. Standard Meals: Moms who miss meals may get grumpy and exhausted. Regular breakfast, lunch, and supper eating schedules maintain consistent energy levels throughout the day.

Moms feel better, more confident, and more equipped to face the day when they eat a healthy diet!

8.2 Easy and Quick Dinners: Healthful Selections for Active Schedules

Moms might get so busy at times that it seems hard to prepare a large lunch. However, there are many quick and simple meals that are nourishing as well:

1. Smoothies: To make a tasty and nutritious smoothie, blend fruits, vegetables, yogurt, and a small amount

of milk or juice. It's convenient and quick to sip on the go.

2. Salad Jars: Arrange chicken, beans, veggies, and a small amount of dressing in a jar. When ready to eat, give it a shake. Similar to a salad on the move!

3. Midnight Breakfast: In a container, combine oats, milk, and a few fruits; refrigerate overnight. It is ready for eating in the morning. It's an excellent, speedy breakfast.

4. Wraps: Roll up veggies, hummus, and lean meats like chicken or turkey on whole wheat tortillas. Similar to a sandwich, but easier to prepare.

5. Stir-Fries: Simmer some vegetables and lean protein with a small amount of soy sauce in a pan. Serve it with quinoa or brown rice for a quick and healthful supper.

Moms can keep energized with these quick and easy meals that provide them with the nutrition they need.

8.3 Successful Meal Planning: Make a Weekly Meal Plan in Ahead of Time

Time and stress can be greatly reduced for busy moms by organizing their meals in advance. It resembles a weekly schedule fit for a superhero! This is how mothers can succeed:

1. Create a Menu: List the meals you want to prepare for the coming week. Knowing what ingredients to buy is made easier by this.

2. Food Purchasing: Moms can prepare a grocery list and shop for everything at once once the menu is finished. They get what they need and save time.

3. Prepare in Groups: Mothers are able to prepare large quantities of food, which they may subsequently portion out for consumption during the week. For instance, prepare a large pot of chili or soup and freeze or refrigerate it.

4. Pre-Cut Vegetables: Moms can chop all the veggies at once and store them in the refrigerator because it takes time to cut them. When needed, they can then be put to use.

5. Apples with Port: To make healthy snacks convenient to grab and go, mothers might split them into little bags or containers.

Eating healthily is a lot easier when meals are prepared, especially on hectic days.

8.4 Stay Hydrated: Maintaining Hydration for Best Results

Water is necessary for an automobile to function correctly, much like fuel is. Our physical selves are identical. It's crucial to stay hydrated, particularly when working out. How can mothers remain hydrated?

1. Always Drink Water: Mothers ought to stay hydrated all day long, not just when they're feeling peckish. Having a water bottle close by aids in reminding children to take frequent sips.

2. Infused Water: Moms can flavor simple water by adding fruit slices, such as lemon, cucumber, or berries.

3. Hydrating Foods: Certain foods contain a lot of water, such as oranges, cucumbers, and watermelon. Consuming them can aid with hydration.

4. Reduce Sugar-Sugary Drinks: Moms may get more

thirsty as a result of drinking beverages like soda and sugary juices. The greatest beverage to stay hydrated is water.

Moms who drink enough water have more energy and perform better during their everyday activities and workouts.

A healthy diet is similar to providing mothers the superpowers they require to manage their hectic schedules. Moms can feel strong and prepared for anything by planning ahead, eating a balanced diet, cooking quick and nourishing meals, and drinking plenty of water. Thus, remember that your mother is fuelling up to be her best self when you see her making a smoothie or sipping water!

CHAPTER 9

Remaining Inspired: Overcoming Obstacles in Your Fitness

9.1 SMART (specific, measurable, attainable, relevant, and time-bound) goal-setting

Envision possessing a treasure map with a large X designating the location of the hidden treasure. Similar to that map, SMART objectives provide moms with step-by-step instructions on how to achieve their fitness treasure!

1. Specific: Mothers ought to have a specific goal in mind. For instance, someone could say, "I want to jog for 20 minutes, three times a week," as opposed to, "I want to exercise more."
2. Metric: Mothers ought to be able to monitor their development. They can track how many workouts they've completed each week using a calendar or a fitness app.

3. Achievable: Mothers should set realistic goals that they can actually accomplish. Moms can succeed by taking little measures at first and then gradually increasing them.

4. Relevant: Moms should have goals that bring them happiness and health. It's comparable to having a goal that has a significant impact.

5. Time-Limited: Mothers should establish a deadline for completing their task. They could state, "By the end of the month, I want to be able to perform 10 push-ups," for instance.

Moms find it simpler to maintain focus and experience pride when they meet their fitness objectives when they set SMART goals.

9.2 Locating a Training Partner: Enlist a Friend or Family Member to Join You on the Adventure

Exercise with friends or family keeps fitness enjoyable and keeps mothers engaged. It seems like you have a teammate supporting you! This is why it's fantastic:

1. Encouragement: Moms who work out with friends can support one another and rejoice in little successes together.

2. Accountability: Moms are more likely to stick to their exercise regimens when they know someone is depending on them. When they know someone is waiting for them, they are less inclined to skip an exercise.

3. Enjoyable Exercises: When mothers have someone to laugh and converse with, exercising feels less like work and more like playtime.

Exercise is more fun when you have a workout partner, be it a friend, your sibling, or even you.

9.3 Monitoring Your Development: Honor Your Successes

Imagine receiving a gold star for every accomplishment in the classroom. That's kind of how tracking progress works; it's about recognizing and applauding all the incredible things mothers accomplish on their fitness journeys!

1. Maintaining a Journal: Moms might journal about their daily workout routines and feelings. Taking a look back at their progress is enjoyable.

2. Determining Benchmarks: Moms ought to rejoice each time they do a task, no matter how tiny! They could buy a new wardrobe for their workout or treat themselves to a movie.

3. Noting Advancements: Moms may monitor their progress and see how much stronger and healthier they are getting. It's similar to getting access to new game levels!

Honoring accomplishments gives mothers the drive and enthusiasm to carry on.

9.4 Overcoming Obstacles: Regaining Focus After Skipping Exercises

It's acceptable when things don't always go as planned! Everyone experiences failures. What counts are the resilience and perseverance of mothers. How can they accomplish it, exactly?

1. Keep Going: Moms shouldn't quit working out completely just because they missed one session. The following day, they can resume their progress and go onward.

2. Grow from Errors: Mothers might reflect on what caused them to skip a workout and devise strategies for avoiding it in the future. Perhaps they can ask for assistance or reschedule their workouts for a different time.

3. Treat Yourself with Love: Everybody experiences difficult days. Mothers ought to be kind to themselves and keep in mind that one failure does not mean that all of their hard work is in vain.

Regaining momentum following a setback is a superpower that enables mothers to continue pursuing their fitness objectives.

To sum up, maintaining motivation requires establishing specific objectives, enlisting the help of others, acknowledging accomplishments, and taking lessons from setbacks. Moms can persevere in their fitness quest by setting SMART objectives, working out with friends, monitoring their progress, and recovering from failures. Therefore, encourage your mother when you see her establishing goals or working out with a friend since she is making incredible efforts to maintain her health and happiness!

CHAPTER 10

REST AND RELAXATION AS SELF-CARE FOR BUSY MOMS

10.1 The Value of Sleep: Recuperate After a hectic day

Think of sleep as the secret power of a superhero. It gives mothers the confidence to face any challenge head-on! This is why getting enough sleep is crucial:

1. Boost Your Energy: Mothers' bodies and minds have an opportunity to relax and rejuvenate when they sleep. Like leaving your phone plugged in to charge all night.

2. Happy Mood: Mothers who get enough sleep are happier and more patient. When they are well-rested, managing hectic days is simpler.

3. Healthy Body: Sleep allows moms' bodies to rebuild and fortify, keeping them healthier.

Moms can try setting a consistent bedtime, reading a book or taking a warm bath, and making sure their bedroom is dark and quiet to help them get enough sleep.

10.2 Mindfulness and Meditation: Stress-Reduction Methods

Moms may feel overpowered by stress, which is like a huge wave. Mothers who practice mindfulness and meditation can ride the wave more peacefully, much like surfboards. This is how they function:

1. Creativity: Focusing on the here and now is one way that mothers can engage in mindfulness practices. They can pay attention to their breathing or their physical sensations. It keeps them composed and concentrated.

2. Tranquility: It's as if you're giving their minds a peaceful vacation. Mothers are able to sit quietly, close their eyes, and reflect on calm topics. It's similar to pausing a hectic day.

These methods assist mothers in reducing stress, increasing relaxation, and improving decision-making.

10.3 Paying Attention to Your Body: Take Breaks When Needed

Think of your body as a friend that lets you know when it needs a vacation. Mothers ought to pay attention to their bodies' needs and provide for them. This is the reason it matters:

1. Recovery and Rest: Mothers get fatigued or sore sometimes. Their body is communicating that it needs to rest. Moms who take a break are better able to handle their next workout or hectic day.
2. Health Indications: Mothers ought to be aware of any discomfort or suffering. It's acceptable to seek medical assistance or take a break till one feels better.

Mothers maintain their health and happiness by paying attention to their bodies.

10.4 Scheduling Time for Yourself: Plan Fun Activities for Yourself

Although mothers give so much to others, it's crucial that they also pursue their passions. The following justifies mothers taking time for themselves:

1. Hobbies and Fun: Mothers can plan time for hobbies and pastimes such as reading, painting, or taking walks in the outdoors. It promotes their happiness and relaxation.

2. Social Time: It's also crucial to spend time with loved ones. Moms can schedule phone conversations or get-togethers to laugh and catch up.

3. Taking Care of Yourself: Giving themselves a small treat is what it means to do activities that make moms feel good, like doing yoga, getting a haircut, or having a bubble bath.

Moms who look for themselves have more love and energy to devote to their family.

As a whole, self-care is akin to providing mothers the abilities they require to continue being strong and content. Moms can take care of themselves in a number of ways, including getting enough sleep, engaging in mindfulness and meditation, paying attention to their bodies, and scheduling time for hobbies and interests. Thus, remember that your mother is taking care of herself so she may be the best mother she can be for you when you see her unwinding or doing something she enjoys!

ABOUT THE AUTHOR

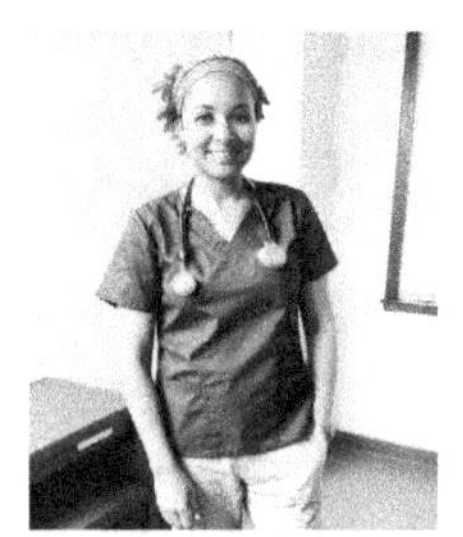 Harmony Royce is a dedicated healthcare worker who has a strong interest in holistic wellness. Harmony's extensive history in various aspects of health and wellness provides her with a wealth of knowledge and expertise that she can utilize in her writing and professional endeavors.

Harmony is a talented author who crafts thought-provoking books that inspire readers to have well-rounded, balanced lives. She writes about a variety of health-related topics, such as diet, exercise, mental health, and mindfulness. Her approachable writing style combines practical guidance with evidence-based research to make complex health concepts approachable and engaging for readers of all ages.

Harmony actively promotes the benefits of holistic health through writing, community workshops, and internet forums. Her mission is to educate and inspire people about the transformative power of self-care and healthy lifestyle choices.

www.ingramcontent.com/pod-product-compliance
Lightning Source LLC
Chambersburg PA
CBHW051659250726
48653CB00007B/2752